Key Strategies for Co-parenting

Co-parenting with a Narcissistic Ex

Robert P. Wright

Table of Contents

Introduction

co-parenting with an egotistical former partner. Any divorced parent would get tired just reading that sentence. It's a never-ending nightmare to deal with a manipulative, demanding, and self-absorbed ex, particularly when kids are involved. The stability of your family dynamic, your mental peace of mind, and your children's well-being all hang in the balance.

The good news is that you have more influence than you may think in this circumstance. Even in situations when you feel helpless, you may regain control by using tried-and-true methods to establish limits, deal with manipulation, and regain your power. You may also decrease conflict and protect your children from long-term damage by putting important parenting techniques into practice.

You'll find a step-by-step guide to handling co-parenting difficulties with assurance and competence in this book. I'll provide you with professional insight into the narcissistic ex's psyche and arm you with defence mechanisms for both your children and yourself. You'll gain knowledge on subjects like:

> How to recognize and comprehend narcissistic actions so that you may react appropriately

➢ Establishing and upholding boundaries with clarity to preserve self-care

➢ Using alternative parenting strategies to avoid drama

➢ Acknowledging the typical manipulative techniques they use on you and the children

➢ Building emotional fortitude during trying circumstances

By adhering to these useful suggestions, which are supported by psychological research and genuine client case studies, you will be able to regain control over your ex's damaging behaviours. Additionally, you'll be prepared to thoughtfully explain the issue to your children.

Keep this horror from continuing. Learn the essential tactics to resist your ex's manipulation and have a pleasant co-parenting relationship. With this book, you regain control over your destiny.

Chapter One

Understanding Narcissistic Personality
Disorder

What is NPD, first of all? It's a disease that causes individuals to believe that they are the most significant and amazing person in the world and that everyone else exists just for their admiration and freedom to do as they like. It sounds awesome, doesn't it? Who wouldn't desire that kind of feeling? Not quite so quickly, however. There's a catch. In actuality, people with NPD are very insecure and have poor self-esteem. They are unable to tolerate rejection or criticism and want continuous affirmation and attention to feel good about themselves. In addition, they struggle to understand other people's emotions and often take advantage of or manipulate others to achieve their goals. It's not all fun and games, as you can see. It's a lonely and painful way to live.

So how can one determine if a person has NPD? Well, there are a few commonplace actions and mindsets that may help you figure it out. People who have NPD, for instance, may:

1. Exaggerate or falsify their accomplishments, skills, appearance, or belongings to justify their excessive boasting.
2. Act arrogant and despise anyone they perceive to be less significant or unique than themselves.

3. Expect others to follow their wishes without questioning them and demand special treatment from others.

4. Show extreme sensitivity and resentment when they don't get the recognition or acclaim they believe they are due.

5. Feel that they are destined for greatness and have aspirations of becoming wealthy, powerful, famous, or flawless.

6. Feel envious of those who possess what they want and assume that others share their feelings.

7. Be very self-centred and only consider their own needs and desires, not those of others.

8. Have no empathy, sympathy, or regret for the people they have harmed.

It does sound like a nightmare. It does get worse. People with NPD also struggle greatly with parenting and relationships. They often alienate and harm the people closest to them, such as their family, friends, or lovers, since they are so egocentric and insensitive. They might:

A. Exert extreme control and abuse, demanding that their spouses or kids comply with their every request.

B. Be very dishonest and disloyal, lying to their kids or cheating on their relationships.

C. Show extreme disregard and indifference, ignoring the needs and emotions of their spouses or kids.

D. Be very jealous and competitive, often attempting to outdo their spouse or kids in anything they do.

E. Have very high expectations for their spouses or children that they are unable to satisfy; they tend to be quite unrealistic and demanding.

As you might guess, these actions often result in confrontations, fights, breakups, or divorces, as well as significant harm and suffering to their loved ones. Since people with NPD are often seen by others as haughty, impolite, or bothersome, they may also find it difficult to sustain friendships, professional ties, or social engagements.

Thus, how may those with NPD be assisted? So, admitting they have a problem and getting expert assistance is the first step. This is challenging since individuals with NPD often don't believe they are defective and may even assign responsibility for their problems to others. However, individuals may gain from psychotherapy, a kind of talk therapy that can assist them in understanding their condition and altering their behaviour, provided they are prepared to acknowledge that they need assistance. Psychotherapy is beneficial to them because:

1) Learn to see the positives and negatives of people and oneself, and

cultivate a more realistic and balanced perspective of both.

2) Develop more self-worth and self-compassion, as well as discover coping mechanisms for their insecurities and shame.

3) Develop their communication and empathy abilities, as well as their understanding of and regard for the needs and emotions of others.

4) Control their feelings and inclinations, and develop constructive coping mechanisms for rejection and criticism.

5) Learn to appreciate the process rather than simply the result, and set reasonable and attainable objectives.

In addition, psychotherapy may assist them in addressing any other mental health conditions they may be experiencing since NPD patients often struggle with despair, anxiety, and drug misuse.

Chapter Two

Setting Boundaries

In a relationship, boundaries are the restrictions you place on both yourself and other people. They support you in safeguarding your health, honouring your needs and morals, and keeping others from abusing or harming you. Setting limits is particularly important when working with an ex-partner who exhibits narcissism, since they may have a mistaken sense of entitlement, self-importance, and empathy deficit.

Establishing boundaries with a narcissistic ex-partner has many advantages:

a. You can go on with your life and recover from the relationship.

b. Unnecessary drama, conflict, and tension may be avoided.

c. You can lessen the possibility that your ex may manipulate, mistreat, or take advantage of you.

d. You can boost your confidence and sense of self-worth.

e. You have the power to cultivate better bonds with both others and yourself.

Here are a few examples of limits you may want to think about:

Communication boundaries:
These are the guidelines you establish for why, how, and when you speak with your former partner. For instance, you may

choose to restrict the amount, timing, and manner of communication, or to limit your conversation to certain subjects like kids or money. If your ex is bothering you, being abusive, or sending you useless emails or messages, you may also decide to block or ignore them.

Time boundaries:

These are the guidelines you establish for how much time you and your children spend together, or how much time you spend with your ex. For instance, you could choose to only meet in public spaces or to avoid meeting your ex. You may also arrange for a third party to mediate the handover, or you can establish a timetable for when your ex can pick up or see the kids.

Physical boundaries:

These are the limits you establish on the amount of closeness or physical contact you have with your ex, as well as the amount of time they may spend with you or your kids. You could choose, for instance, to decline any unwanted hugs, kisses, or physical contact, as well as to forgo any romantic or sexual activity with your former partner.

Emotional boundaries:

These are the guidelines you establish for how much you listen to or care about your ex's emotions, thoughts, or views, as well as how much you share your feelings, thoughts, or ideas with them. For instance, you may choose to refrain from arguing or debating with your ex and just have factual, impersonal chats. You may also decide not to allow your ex's feelings to influence your choices or your attitude by separating yourself from them.

Now, how can these limits be regularly and gently enforced? Now, the following advice could be useful to you:

Be firm and explicit with your ex:
Let them know what your limits are, why you value them, and what will happen if they are crossed. Make use of "I" phrases like "I need you to respect my privacy and stop calling me at night", and "I will not tolerate any insults or threats from you". Avoid being evasive, unclear, or contrite.

Remain strong and consistent:

Don't let your ex coerce, shame-trip, or threaten you into adjusting your limits. Instead, stand by them. Refuse to budge by their threats, entreaties, or assurances. Don't accept their actions as an exception or an explanation. Avoid giving conflicting messages or being contradictory.

Act civil and courteous:

Show your ex-partner decency and civility, and anticipate the same in return. Avoid being impolite, antagonistic, or violent. Never make fun of, disparage, or offend them. Avoid accusing, humiliating, and calling names. Avoid taking vengeance or retaliating.

Be flexible and realistic:

Acknowledge that your limits may not be ideal and that you might need to modify them as circumstances change. As long as suggestions are sensible and kind, be willing to listen and make concessions. Avoid being inflexible, obstinate, or unreasonable.

Chapter Three

Parallel Parenting Approaches

When you and your ex are at odds and don't get along, one approach to raising your kids after a divorce or separation is via parallel parenting. In contrast to co-parenting, which entails regular communication and teamwork, parallel parenting entails solo parenting and little contact with your former partner. As long as they are not damaging or abusive, you each have the right to establish your guidelines, practices, and judgments for your kids.

You may be wondering why co-parenting with a high-conflict ex is preferable to parallel parenting. Thus, the following are a few advantages of parallel parenting:

1. Both you and your kids experience less stress and anxiety as a result. You don't have to put up with your ex's persistent fights, disputes, or insults. You may provide your kids with a secure and tranquil atmosphere while concentrating on your pleasure and well-being.

2. It shields your kids from the damaging impacts of parental disagreement. The animosity, stress, or violence that might arise between you and your former partner is not something you expose your kids to. You don't include your kids in your arguments or give

them the impression that they have to choose a side or appease you both. You don't use your kids as couriers or spies, nor do you disparage or criticize each other in front of them.

3. It makes it possible for your kids to get along well with both of you. You value your children's rights and acknowledge their need for your affection as much as your own. You don't attempt to keep your children apart from your ex or meddle with their parenting time. You encourage your kids to enjoy their time with both of you and support their relationship with your ex.

So, what is the secret to successful parallel parenting? So, the following recommendations should help to ease stress and enhance coordination:

Draft a comprehensive and targeted parenting strategy. This written document contains all of the plans you have for your kids, including the timetable, holidays, vacations, schooling, health care, extracurricular activities, and communication. Confusion and disagreement are less likely to arise in a strategy that is more precise and well-defined. To assist you in developing a strategy that benefits you and your kids, you may consult a lawyer, a mediator, or an internet resource.

Adhere to the parenting schedule consistently. Once you've made a plan, follow it through without straying unless both of you agree otherwise or there's an emergency. You shouldn't make adjustments without first talking to your ex or assuming that they would comply with your wishes. Don't attempt to increase or decrease your ex's parenting time, be late, or cancel your parenting time. Never introduce new partners or make big life changes to your kids without first telling your former spouse.

Only speak when required and do so with decency. Refrain from speaking with your ex over the phone or in person since this might lead to conflict or negative feelings. To stay in touch with each other regarding significant matters concerning your kids, such as their health, school, or special occasions, use text messaging, email, or an app like Our Family Wizard. Communicate in a succinct, factual, and courteous manner. Avoid making accusations, insults, or sarcasm. Don't talk about your private life, your emotions, or your thoughts about your former partner.

Lastly, how do you maintain your composure during boring talks regarding the kids? Here are some pointers to assist you, then:

1. Pay attention to the here and now rather than the past. Don't discuss past transgressions, errors, or regrets. Don't hold your ex accountable for

your relationship's problems or pass judgment on them. Don't make an effort to influence, persuade, or alter your ex. Recognize that you cannot alter your ex-partner; they are who they are. Give the past a shot and move on with your life.

2. Establish limits and boundaries with your ex. Keep your ex from going too far or infringing on your rights. Refrain from allowing your former partner to coerce, threaten, or induce guilt into doing actions against your will. Keep your ex out of your life and don't allow them to intrude on your private. When necessary, say no, and advocate for yourself. If your former partner is acting disrespectfully or

abusively, don't hesitate to cut off communication or ban them.

3. Ask for assistance and support as required. Avoid attempting to manage everything by yourself. Seek out financial, practical, or emotional help from friends, family, or a support group. Speak with a coach, therapist, or counsellor for expert direction and help. Seek out constructive outlets for your stress, such as physical activity, meditation, or hobbies. Make sure you look after yourself and pursue your happiness.

Chapter Four

Managing Potential Manipulation

In a nutshell, manipulation tactics are deceptive and covert methods of moulding or manipulating the thoughts, feelings, or actions of another person. Manipulators often exhibit a delusional feeling of entitlement, self-importance, and empathy deficits. Additionally, they could be more likely to influence people if they have a personality problem like narcissistic personality disorder (NPD).

What are some typical strategies of manipulation used by narcissistic ex-partners? There are a lot, but here are a few of the more common ones:

Gaslighting:

This is the practice of lying, denying, or distorting the truth to get you to question your reality or recollection. Says like "You're crazy, that never happened," "You're too sensitive, I was just joking," or "You're the one who started the fight, not me" are a few examples of what they could say.

Love bombing:

This occurs when someone shows you an excessive amount of love, gifts, attention, or praise, often when the relationship is just getting started or after a fight. They could remark something like, "You're the only person who understands me," "You're the best thing that has ever happened to me," or "I can't live without you."

Triangulation:

This is the process by which they instigate conflict, envy, or insecurity by creating or using a third party, such as a friend, relative, or former spouse. They could say something like, "My mom says you're not good enough for me," "My friend thinks you're too controlling," or "My ex still loves me, you know."

Guilt-tripping:

This occurs when someone makes you feel as if you are to blame for their moods, behaviours, or issues. Says like "You're the reason I'm unhappy," "If you loved me, you would do this for me," or "You owe me for everything I've done for you" are a few examples of what they could say.

Lying:

This is when someone gives you incorrect or misleading information to trick you, shift the responsibility, or accomplish their goals. Sayings like "I worked late, I swear," "I didn't cheat on you, I swear," or "I borrowed your money instead of spending it" are a few examples of what someone may say.

Flattery:

This is when someone gives you undeserved or excessive compliments in an attempt to control you, win your confidence, or get an advantage over you. Says like "You're so smart, you can do anything," "You're so beautiful, you don't need makeup," or "You're so generous, you can lend me some money" are a few examples of what they could say.

Projection:
This is the accusation that you share their shortcomings, emotions, or motivations. "You're the one who's selfish, not me," "You're the one who's insecure, not me," or "You're the one who's cheating, not me" are a few examples of what they could say.

Emotional blackmail:
This occurs when someone threatens to harm you, themselves, or a third party if you refuse to comply with their demands. They could say things like, "I'll kill myself if you leave me," "I'll tell everyone your secrets if you don't give me another chance," or "I'll cut you off from our friends if you don't agree with me."

Victim playing:

This occurs when someone, even if they are the ones who started the issue, presents themselves as the defenceless, naive, or misunderstanding victim of another person's actions. They can say things like, "You don't understand how much I suffer because of you," "You don't understand how hard my life is," or "You don't appreciate how much I sacrifice for you."

It sounds familiar, doesn't it? You're not alone, so don't worry. These deception techniques have been used on a large number of individuals at some time in their lives. The good news is that you can develop the ability to identify them and defend yourself against them. The following techniques may be used to spot manipulation:

Follow your instincts:
If anything seems strange, incorrect, or too good to be true, it most likely is. Don't allow your emotions or instincts to influence your decisions. Keep an eye out for any warning signs or contradictions in their statements and behaviour.

Educate yourself:
Get as much knowledge as you can on narcissistic personality disorder, manipulative techniques, and other relevant subjects. Your ability to recognize manipulation's telltale indications and patterns will increase with knowledge. A therapist, counsellor, or coach may also

provide you with professional guidance and support.

Make inquiries:

Do not accept their words at face value. Test them, ask them questions, and put their assertions to the test. Never hesitate to request a proof, elucidation, or an explanation. Don't let them sidestep, divert, or alter the topic. You shouldn't allow them to make you feel foolish, guilty, or insane for posing inquiries.

Request feedback:

Avoid isolating yourself or depending just on your viewpoint. Speak with your loved ones, friends, or other reliable individuals who can provide you with frank and unbiased criticism. Find out what they think of your spouse, your relationship, and their actions. Even if their thoughts vary from your own, pay attention to their advice and ideas.

Maintain a record:

Jot down or document any discussions, occurrences, or occasions involving manipulation. Note down the times, dates, locations, and individuals who are involved. Regularly go over your records and search for any trends, inconsistencies, or disparities. This may assist you in maintaining your sense of reality, avoiding confusion, and remembering the facts.

And lastly, how do you react without getting sucked into the drama? Here are a few methods for achieving that:

Establish limits:

Choose what actions, behaviours, and levels of tolerance you are and are not willing to accept in a relationship. Adhere to your boundaries with assertiveness and clarity. Keep them from going too far or infringing on your rights. Refrain from allowing them to coerce, threaten, or induce guilt into altering your boundaries.

Remain composed:

Avoid allowing them to irritate, provoke, or get under your skin. Avoid having an impulsive, defensive, or emotional reaction. Avoid having discussions, arguments, or drama. Don't encourage their dramatization or negativity. Remain cool, collected, and polite. If necessary, take a deep breath, count to ten, or get up and move on.

Be reasonable:
Don't anticipate an apology, change, or admission of guilt from them. Refuse to accept their excuses, lies, or promises. Make no excuses for them, don't sympathize with them, or idealize them. Recognize them for who they are and accept the circumstances as they are. Be not gullible, naive, or optimistic. Be cautious, sceptical, and realistic.

Detach yourself:
Don't let them control you, influence you, or affect you. Refrain from giving them your time, effort, or focus. Don't let them interfere with your life, goals, or happiness.

Never rely on them, never have faith in them, and never show them any concern. Detach yourself from them emotionally, mentally, and physically.

Seek help:

Don't try to deal with them alone. Consult your loved ones, friends, or other dependable individuals for assistance in coping, healing, and moving on. Consult with a coach, therapist, or counsellor who can assist you in comprehending, processing, and healing from the manipulation. Seek help from a lawyer, police, or other authorities if you are in danger, abused, or harassed.

Chapter Five

Taking Care of Yourself

What does self-care entail? It's the act of looking after your whole health—physical, mental, emotional, and spiritual. It's not conceited, frivolous, or indolent. It's fulfilling, empowering, and necessary. It's how you treat yourself with kindness, love, and respect. It's how you rejuvenate yourself, elevate your state of mind, and enhance your life.

Now, why is self-care crucial, particularly in this circumstance? Here are a few of the causes, though:

It facilitates good stress management. Stress is unavoidable, particularly if your narcissistic ex is causing you a lot of drama, conflict, or hurt. Yet stress may also be detrimental to your performance, happiness, and health. The negative consequences of stress, such as anxiety, sadness, sleeplessness, or disease, may be lessened, managed, or prevented with the use of self-care.

It facilitates your recovery from the abuse and trauma. Abuse and trauma are grave problems that may have an impact on your health, mind, and spirit. They have the power to make you feel numb, furious, afraid, or sad. They may also undermine your trust, confidence, and sense of self. Taking care of yourself may aid in your recovery from whatever injuries and scars your former partner may have caused you, as well as help you regain confidence, security, and hope.

You can concentrate on your needs and requirements alone. If you're in a relationship with a narcissist, you may have put your ex's wants and happiness above your own. You could no longer recognize yourself, your identity, or your mission. Reestablishing a connection with yourself and your needs, as well as rediscovering your identity, desires, and worth, may be achieved via self-care.

So, how do you take care of yourself? There are several approaches, but here are a few of the more popular ones:

Take care of your body:

You should treat your body with compassion and respect since it is your temple. Eat healthily, stay hydrated, exercise, get enough sleep, and relax. Steer clear of anything that might impair your emotions or health, such as alcohol and narcotics. Give yourself a manicure, a bath, or a massage. Wear what makes you feel good about yourself and at ease.

Take care of your mind:

You must maintain a positive and keen mind since it is your greatest asset. Play a game, watch a movie, read a book, or learn something new. Put yourself through a test, let your imagination run wild, or just share your ideas. Steer clear of unfavourable ideas, influences, or thoughts that might diminish your pleasure or sense of self-worth. Use affirmations, gratitude, or meditation.

Attend to your feelings:
Your feelings are a guide that you should respect and pay attention to. Don't criticize, repress, or reject your sentiments; just be aware of how you are feeling. Laugh, cry, yell, or let it out. Seek solace, consolation, or affirmation from other people. Steer clear of manipulative, abusive, or poisonous persons who might harm or arouse your emotions. Practice compassion, acceptance, or forgiveness.

Look after your soul:

Your spirit is your essence; you must connect with and tend to it. Engage in activities that provide you joy, fulfilment, or inspiration. Achieve your objectives, follow your passion, or follow your dreams. Discover your goal, purpose, or meaning. Make a connection with music, art, nature, or religion. Engage in acts of compassion, charity, or service.

Chapter Six

Conclusion

Co-parenting refers to the collaborative parenting of children by unmarried or divorced parents. Co-parents may never have married or be divorced. They are not romantically involved with one another. Joint parenting is another name for co-parenting. Co-parents collaborate on significant choices concerning their children's development, including those regarding education, healthcare, religious education, and other significant issues, in addition to the usual child care.

Co-parenting may provide your kids with a feeling of consistency, security, and stability, which is good for them. Additionally, it may shield children from the damaging impacts of parental disagreement and help them grow up with a strong connection with both of you. Co-parenting may be difficult, however, particularly if you and your ex often argue, are bitter, or are hostile towards one another. To make it work, you must so adhere to certain co-parenting techniques. These are a few of the more significant ones:

1. Prioritize your kids: This is the most important co-parenting tip. Regardless of your feelings for one another or what transpired between you and your ex, you must put your kids' interests and welfare ahead of your own. Keep your problems out of the way of your parenting duties. Don't use your kids as weapons, pawns, or

messengers to get even with your former partner. Don't force your kids to choose sides or feel bad for loving you both. Avoid disparaging your former partner in front of your kids or undermining their authority or bond with them.

2. Communicate effectively: excellent co-parenting depends on excellent communication. Discussing your children's schedule, health, education, activities, and any other pertinent matters with your former partner is essential. Along with talking to them about the co-parenting schedule, you should also pay attention to their worries and sentiments. Be kind, cooperative, and explicit in your communication. Avoid blaming, criticizing, or arguing. Don't talk about the past or your

issues. To keep track of your correspondence and prevent misunderstandings, use text, email, or an app like Our Family Wizard.

3. Be both flexible and consistent: Co-parenting necessitates striking a balance between the two. Your co-parenting plan may need to be modified in response to unforeseen circumstances, crises, or special events, so you must be adaptable. Additionally, you must be reliable enough to stick to the schedule and honour the guidelines and customs that you and your former partner have established. Don't make changes without first talking to your ex-partner, and don't assume that they will either. Don't attempt to increase or decrease your ex's parenting time, be late, or cancel

your parenting time. Never introduce new partners or make big life changes to your kids without first telling your former spouse.

4. Encourage one another: You must encourage one another as co-parents since parenting is a team endeavour. As long as your ex's parenting methods do not endanger or abuse your kids, you should accept their choices, parenting styles, and viewpoints. Instead of opposing or undermining your ex's rules and penalties, you should support them. It's important that you support your kids' healthy and happy connection with your ex and don't get in the way of their quality time together. As a co-parent, you must respect and value your ex's accomplishments and efforts; do not minimize or take them for granted.

These are some of the most important co-parenting techniques that may support you and your former partner in cooperating to provide your kids with the finest environment possible.

Finally, let me clarify that although co-parenting is feasible, it is not simple. It is worth the time, patience, and work that it could need. As a co-parent, you are doing an excellent job, and you need to be proud of yourself. On this trip, you are not alone. If you need assistance, don't hesitate to ask friends, family, or experts for it. Recall that co-parenting is about your children and their happiness, not about you and your ex.